I0429819

How To Stop Eating Foods You Are Addicted To

in 24 Hours Or Less

Tough

But Guaranteed

By Sophie Johnson

ISBN 13: 9781499508697

ISBN 10: 1499508697

CONTENTS

Sophie Johnson

DEDICATION

This book is dedicated to the memory of my Mum, we dieted together and stayed overweight together, she would have loved this method.

Our high spot was attending Weight Watchers and then getting chips on the way home, after all we had a whole week to lose it.

CHAPTER 1 **STOP**

Before you go any further.

From Sophie Johnson

WARNING:

Please <u>do not read</u> this book unless you *<u>truly</u>* want to stop eating whatever food it is that you are addicted to. *NOT* FOR PREGNANCY CRAVINGS. NOR IF YOU ARE ILL.

Ok, that said, on we go – if you are sure.
This book is short
- but it is lethal to addictive food cravings.

(Remember, **not** if you are pregnant **nor** if you are not in good health, save this for after and please read Publisher's Notes on page 3.

CHAPTER 2 WHO AM I?

My name is Sophie Johnson and I am a Mum of two grown up children both of whom are slim.

I used to be slim but over the years the weight crept on, I hardly noticed as I was busy with life and family. Husband didn't seem to mind having a more cuddly wife and I had lots of excuses to let myself off the hook.

Until came that shocking moment, yes there is always a moment isn't there? For me it was the classic catching sight of myself in a shop window reflection, who was that fat woman staring back at me.

Have you experienced this moment of horror at how you look? A photo taken unawares maybe or a chance remark from someone?

I feel for you. Next step of course is to get on to the diet roundabout, I was determined and for the following 20 plus years I tried them all, probably you have too.

Guess what? Nothing worked for very long, back I would go to being overweight, depressed and cross with myself. Then a moment of clarity seemed to jump into my mind and I couldn't get rid of it.

What luck, what a blessing that moment was. It showed me that I was simply sabotaging all my diet efforts by desperately stuffing myself with an addictive, fatty, weight inducing food. Yes! with crisps!

Why ever would I do this to myself?

Do you do it to yourself with some addictive food? You want it and you don't.

If your answer is yes, then I feel sure that deep down you know why you do it, I did.

Any time some uncomfortable thoughts came up, emotions I didn't want to feel, something I didn't want to face or deal with or even pure boredom, I would reach for the crisps to block everything out. Not consciously of course, I had no idea at the time, but looking back it was so clear.

The end result of my own destructive behaviour around crisps was inevitably that yet another diet bit the dust, more weight seemed to go on each time and I was really miserable again. Ring any bells?

Don't despair, you can fix this kind of self sabotage in double quick time if you are truly ready.

OK, so like me you are addicted to some food or other. For me it has always been crisps, I just can't resist them and they have sabotaged diet after diet and even if they made me feel ill from eating too many, I couldn't stop.

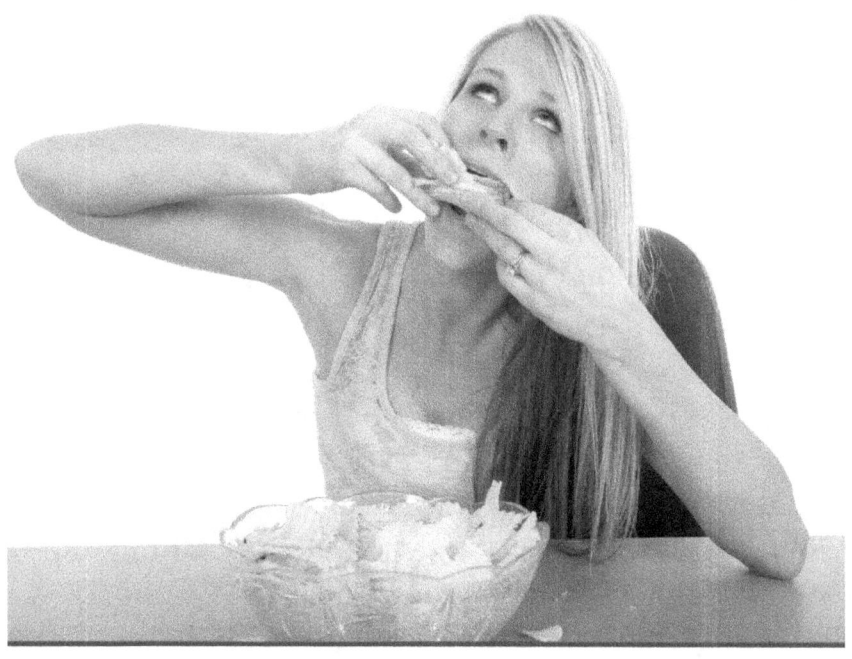

Mmmmm.

I can control my craving for most things, but crisps? Not a chance.

It may be the same for you, is your problem with crisps or some other food that you just can't stop eating? Chips maybe? With salt and vinegar on those crispy little tempters? Or what about oh no, salted peanuts.

Some unlucky souls have a very sweet tooth instead, chocolates, biscuits, cakes, don't worry, this method works for all food addictions.

Whatever the addictive food is for you, you can fix it and fast. I will use crisps as my example.

CHAPTER 3- DO YOU REACH FOR IT?

Even though:

You know it is not good for you.

You know it is sabotaging your diet.

You know you'll regret it later.

You hate yourself every time you reach for it.

I know just how you feel, I hate myself for eating crisps, I eat them whether I am feeling hungry or not, even though I know how it will affect me and my health, kill my diet and make me feel ill and disgusted with myself later on.

Do you go from opening a packet of crisps to an empty bag and not even know what they tasted like nor where they went?

Without even knowing how it happened?

Your craving for crisps and other addictive snacks is adding salt, sugar and tons of fat, ruining your diet and endangering your health.

And there are loads more addictive foods. The manufacturers know all about this in their products and make sure we cannot resist them, they are made that way with sugar, salt and fat to hook us into the product, they call it 'mouth feel' and we fall for those yummy tastes every time.

Bottom line?

If you can't stop eating it, it's a problem.

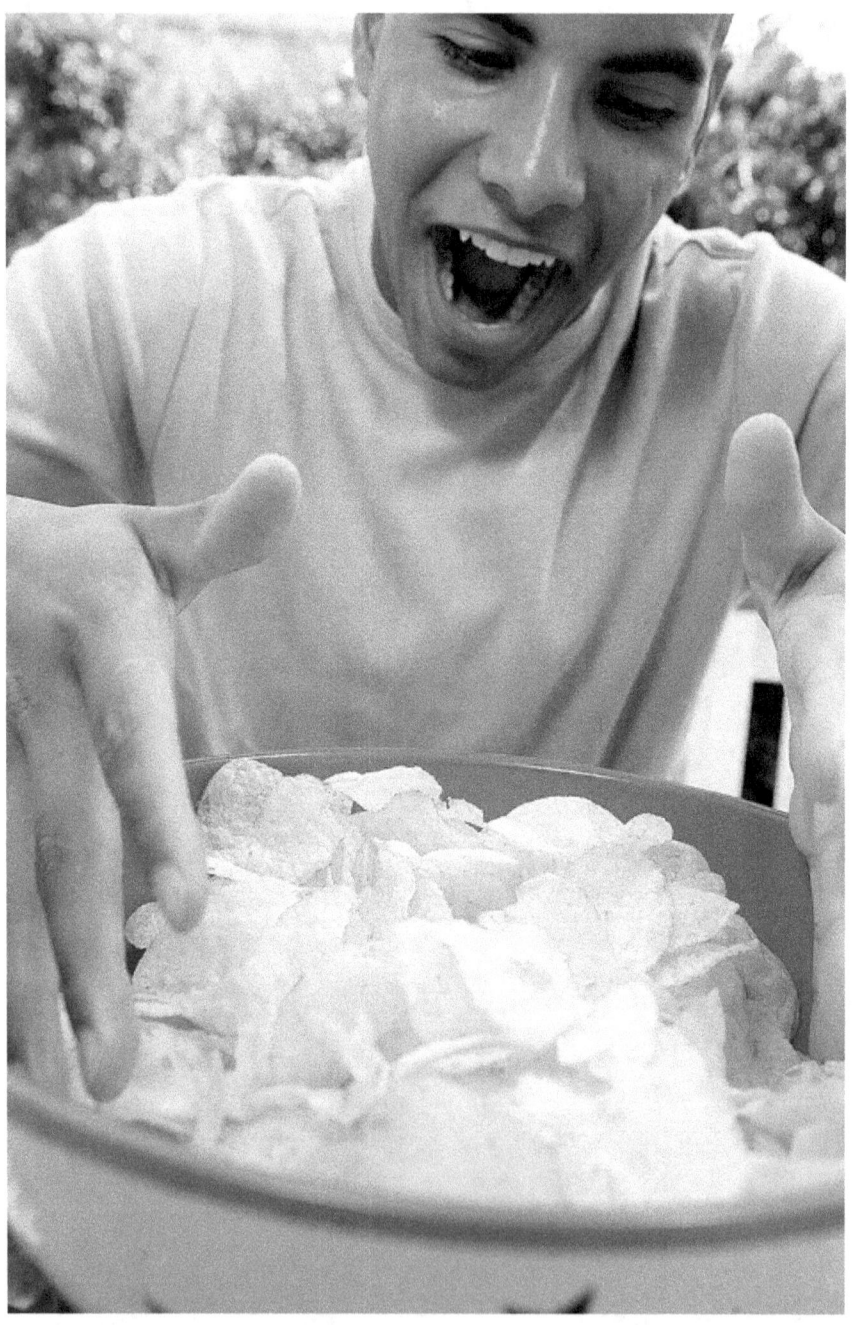

CHAPTER 4- WHAT CAN YOU DO ?

The Usual Advice

Here are some of the usual pieces of advice from well meaning friends and family:

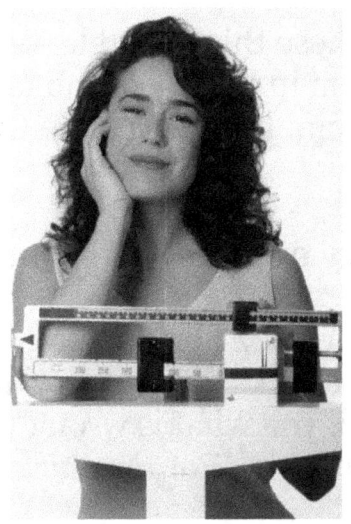

For heaven's sake, just use some will power

Huh, if that works for you then congratulations, it works for me for a while but sooner or later (usually sooner) back I go and the crisps get the upper hand again.

Don't buy it then!

Easy to say and not so easy to do. These addictive foods are everywhere, so easy to drop into a shopping bag, pick up at a corner shop or at work on the trolley.

Then there is 'help' from the family

They **_will_** buy these things and leave them around or even hide them in the house, no matter, I will find them and eat them. I'm worse than the kids if it's crisps!

There is plenty of good sense on websites

Generally about eating healthy food, switching those wonderful salty snacks for celery or an apple. Well I don't need to tell you what is wrong with that advice, good though it may be. For me anyway, it just won't work.

Don't do this unless you really and truly

mean to stop.

CHAPTER 5- SO WHAT WILL WORK?

You need to change the experience of eating your addictive food from a pleasure into pain.

What do I mean by this?

When you eat your addictive food, several things happen. You first of all enjoy the **taste**, particularly the **feel** of it in your mouth, you roll it around and get the **bliss**, especially the **first taste**. Can you feel it now? Mmmm.

You feel fully satisfied, happy, loved. Loved? Wait a minute, how does that come into eating your craved food? The way it makes you feel full, satisfied, safe, is similar to being loved – only similar but enough.

After that it is just downhill, taste? Pah, let's just eat it all, who wants to stop now, who could? Sounds familiar? Thought so.

After the first taste experience things level out a bit, you can eat it all without thinking, without really tasting it any more even.

Then later comes the remorse, the feeling slightly ill if you ate a lot, the recognition that this wasn't such a good idea.

Knowing your diet will fail again because of all the extra, unwanted calories. (You'll see just how many later on, you will be shocked.)

CHAPTER 6- WHAT YOU NEED TO DO

Change the first taste and especially the **texture,** the **FEEL** of the food from your pleasurable friend into something that is **YUK**.

I mean really, really yukky, disgusting, something you would never ever put in your mouth.

The choice of what to change it into will be different for us all but there will be something in your head you can use, you have probably seen the Bushtucker Trials in the Get Me Out Of Here series, that should give you some ideas.

Crunchy squishy mealy bug anyone?

Here we go...

CHAPTER 7- HERE'S HOW TO STOP EATING ADDICTIVE FOODS

For my crisp addiction, when I had finally decided enough was enough, a decision which has taken years I may say. It was when yet another diet failed because I was sabotaging myself with all these extra, useless calories.

(Keep reading if your food addiction is sugar, chocolate and other fatty foods. The method works for all.

This is what I did.

Hating the way I felt after yet another giant pack disappeared, the over full feeling, the feeling of having eaten too much fat, oh it is horrible, but NOT ANY MORE!

You can do this too, easily and forever!

Read on and be free

CHAPTER 8- GET STARTED RIGHT NOW.

(You can do this just for a particular type of salty snack or all of them as well as any sugary or fatty foods.)

For my crisps problem though, I decided to change the crunch of a moreish crisp into the crunch of *live* beetles.

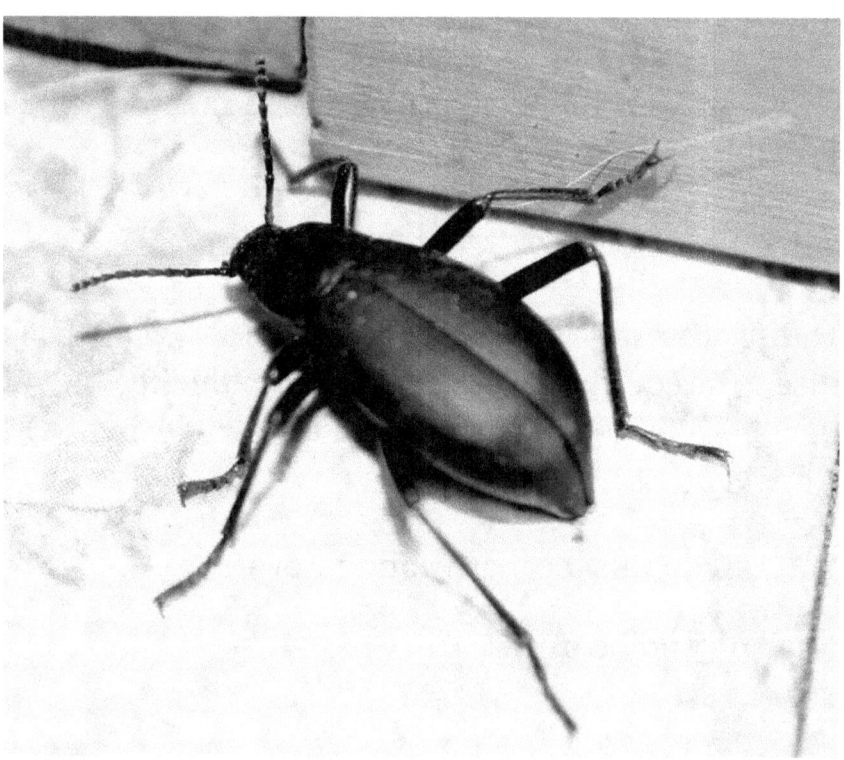

Oh YUK. I imagined their crunchy backs as I bit into them, wings and wriggling legs inside my mouth, on my tongue - instead of the crisp.

Be *ruthless* with your visioning

Important Note: (That means ***IMAGINING*** it, **NOT** actually eating them!)

See images in your mind of the beetles or whatever makes you nearly throw up to think of, *feel it* as you imagine them first going into your mouth, the crunch as you bite into their bodies, beetle shelly backs and their legs wriggling on your tongue.

Oh! Some have WINGS.

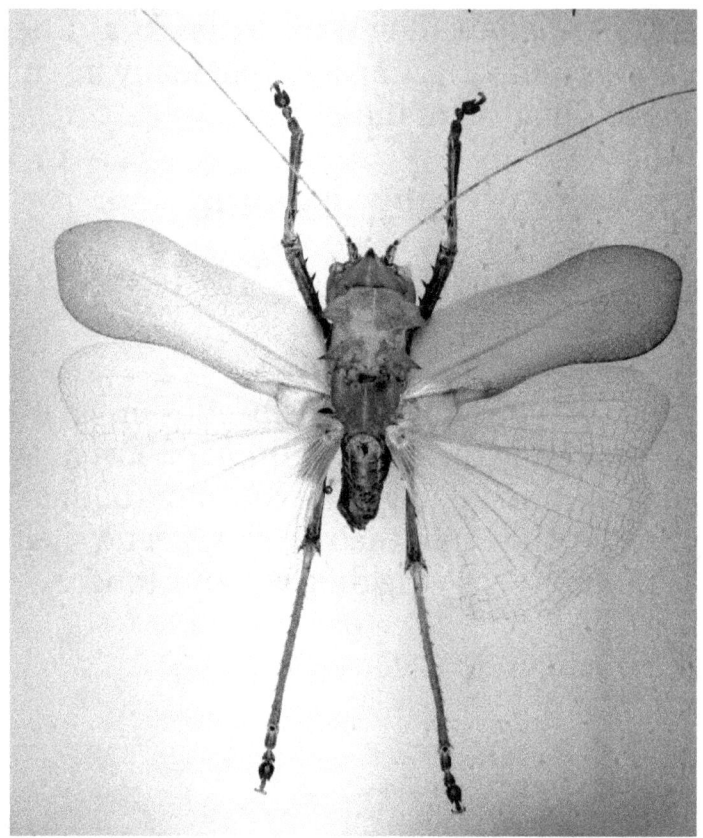

OMG!

<u>Change the experience</u> of eating a crisp, into the mouthful of horrible beetles, *feel* them crunch, hate the strong taste, their wings, their blood and urine as you eat them, as I type this my face is making yuk expressions without me doing it. Probably yours is too, great, this is exactly what we want to happen.

This imagining switch has to be <u>FAST</u>, just like a camera shutter. Click Click.

Think Crisps …. Feel Beetles wriggling in your mouth.

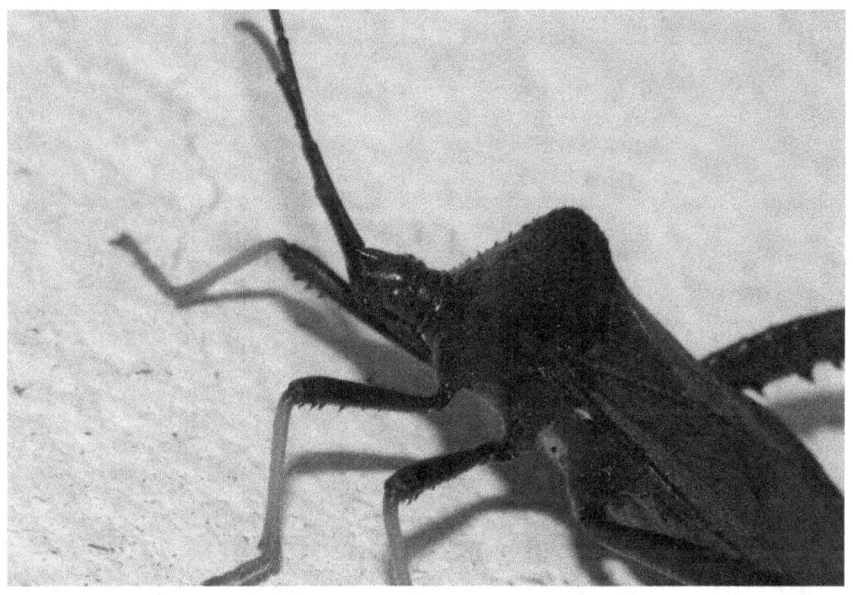

Instantly, no thinking, just switch the images and do it fast   Click, Click.

You have to get it vivid and <u>*every time* - and I mean every single time</u> you think you might just like a crisp,   Click Click. Make the switch instantly, feel the yuk in your mouth.

Do this every single time and *within a day or even less* you will not be able to face eating crisps or whatever your fav salty snack is.

Now, you shouldn't get this far, but if you do ever see yourself dipping into the bag, what will you pull out? Oh no, it's a big horrible cockroach in your

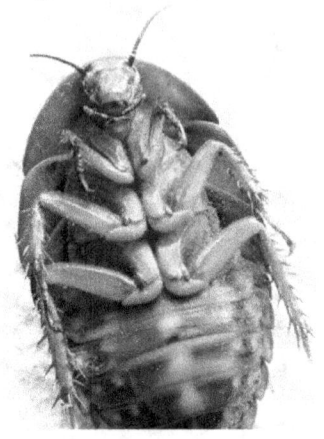

hand, Click Click, strongly imagine putting it in your mouth, immediately feel those beetle shells crunching in your mouth, on your tongue, legs stuck in your teeth. *Double triple yuk.*

If you are not good at seeing the pictures in your mind, really large and bright, then collect some pictures of ghastly things you can hardly bear to look at and paste them on to a board or page to look at when you need to.

Remember, Click, Click

every single time.

Do it fast, without thinking or hesitating.

Make the visioning real, feel it, taste it.

CHAPTER 9- SO TO SUM UP.

Choose a switch which **disgusts** you.
Do you like his feelers? His long legs wriggling on
the roof of your mouth, stuck inbetween your teeth?

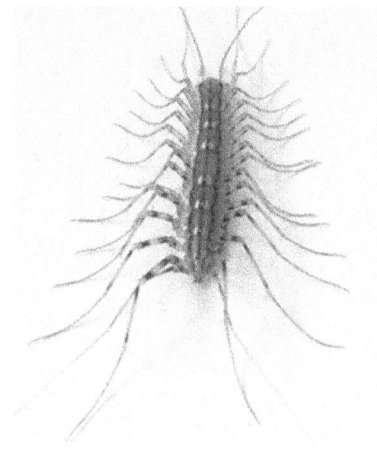

What about some wings? Can you feel them on your
tongue? His furry body? Eeeeugh I know, imagine it
strongly, taste it, feeeeel it.

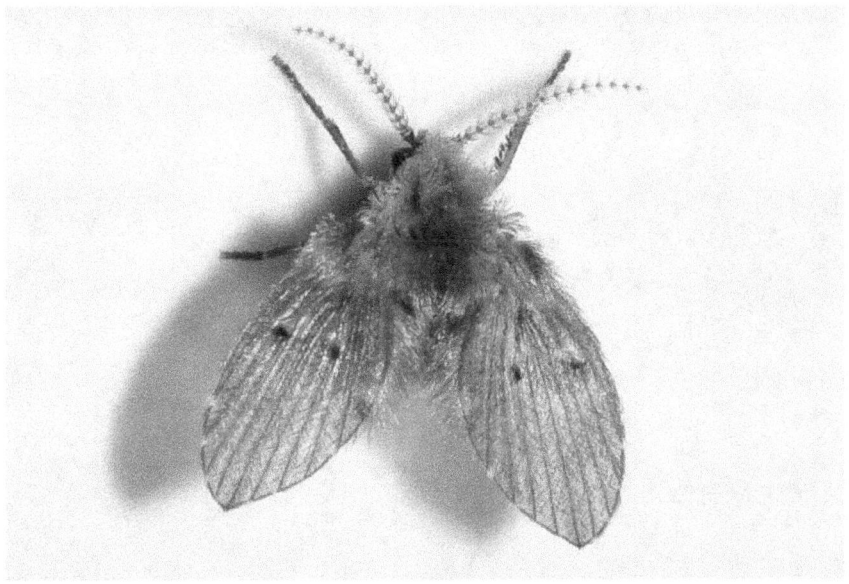

And _especially_ –the crunchy texture.

What would a large, crunchy fly taste like, can you feel its wings, its legs wriggling, the squishy middle, its head and eyes?

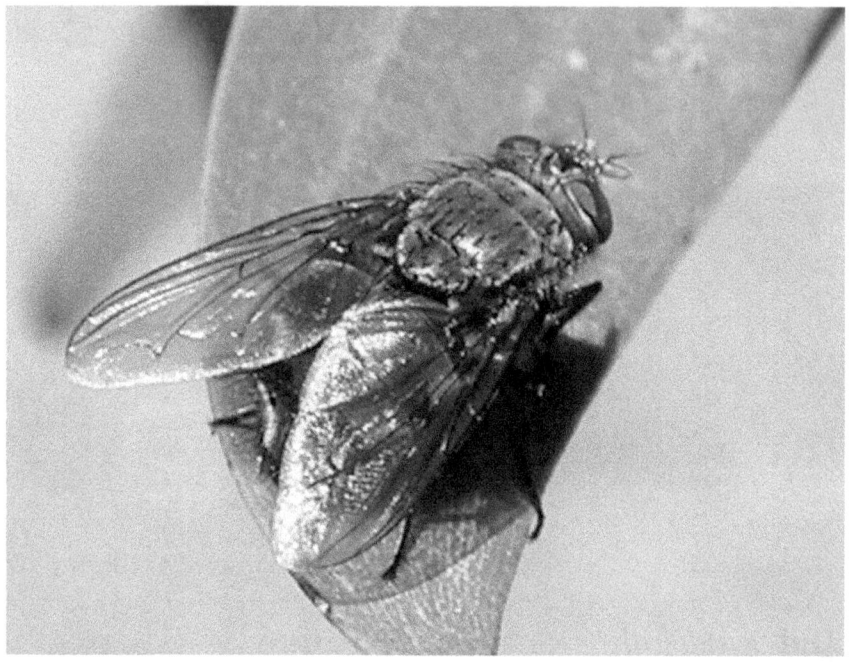

Think of the **experience** of your addictive food and **match** it as best you can, especially the texture, then Click Click switch.

It is up to you, the important things are:-

To choose the replacement to be as bad as you can.

Match it as much as you can to the feel of your addictive food ie the crunch of it or texture of it.

How about a wriggly spider then?

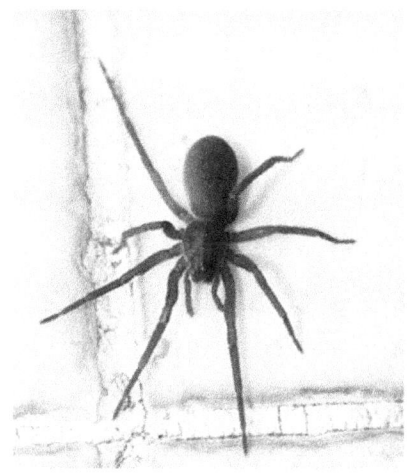

Visualise it as strongly **in your mouth** as you can, *feel it, taste it.*

And always, always, always be *FAST*, Click – Click and switch the images.
As you even think about your addictive food immediately replace the feel, the taste in your mouth with your horrible, disgusting replacement

This cure will work for any food that you are addicted to, change the things you Click Click switch to suit your addictive food.

Chapter 10-Other Addictive Foods Including Chocolate

Chocolate, this is such a common one, I have a friend who would get out of bed, drive to a shop to buy chocolate if she had none in the house. Can you even imagine doing that? Oh, you have!

For your Click Click visualisation may I suggest something that gives that melting, fatty feel on the tongue, what about some nice smooth, tasty engine oil.?

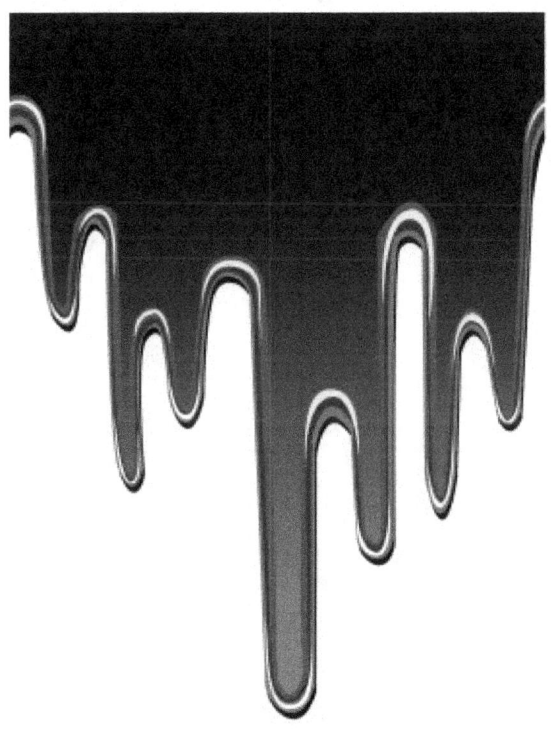

Imagine a mouthful, burnt, acrid and smelling totally horrible, think chocolate Click Click replace it with the visualisation, the feel, of black, gooey, smooth engine oil in your mouth.

If that is not enough, there is something worse that you could visualise, I hesitate to say it, maybe you won't need anything so bad for your cure.

However, if you do, then feel this one on your tongue, sticking to your teeth, coating your lips.

Squash it around your mouth as you Click Click every time you even think about chocolate.

What is it? Why haven't I said?

Well it really is a bad one, so skip over the next page if you don't really want to know. (I've written it small as well)

Yes you guessed it - it's poo.

The texture is perfect and the horror more than enough. If you Click Click this visualisation for chocolate, you are brave and really do want to stop eating that addictive food.

Feel it, smell it, roll it around your teeth, it's sticky and persistant, Click Click.

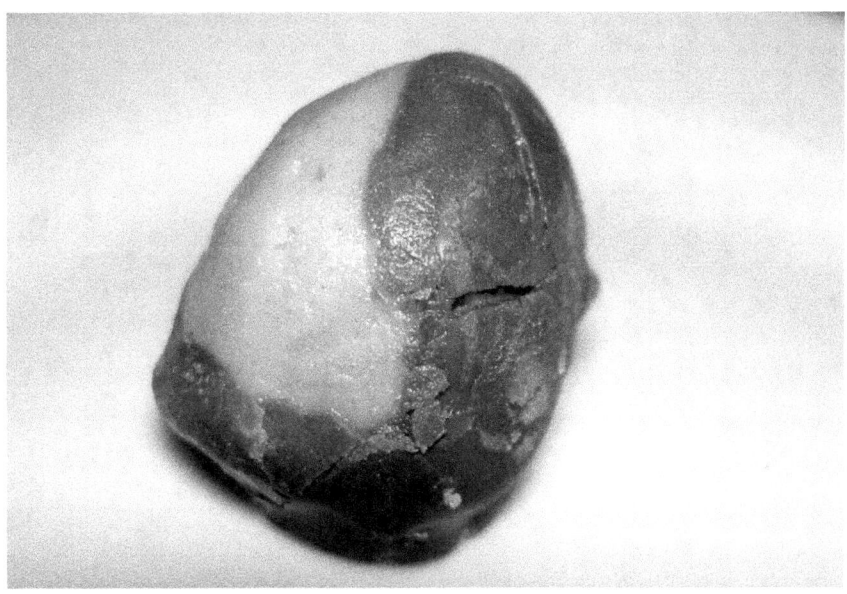

Here is some lovely, gooey chocolate - or is it?

CHAPTER 11- CAKES, BISCUITS ETC.

Are you addicted to cakes I wonder? Or biscuits or sweets maybe?

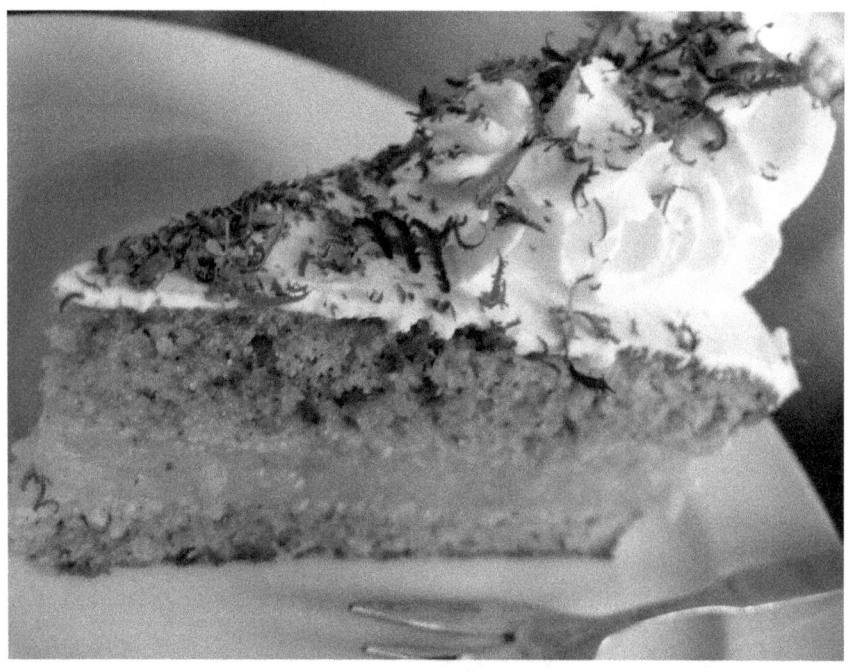

Try switching that creamy scrumptious cake with visualising a Click Click of say biting into a filthy, dirty damp, squidgy old sponge. Or what about mashed up worms mixed with mouldy breadcrumbs?

Biscuits might work if you Click Click with some of the crunchy bugs I used for my crisps addiction.

If you keep visualising it will keep working and far sooner than you can possibly imagine. It will happen in hours, not days or weeks, if you do it right, you will be free.

After a while it will become quite automatic and you won't even have to work at it any more, it will just happen.

I no longer even think about eating crisps even though they are in the house for the grandchildren.

CHAPTER 12 YOUR WONDERFUL GIFTS IN RETURN

Yes, you will receive wonderful gifts in return, check out some of them:

You feel in control and you **_are_** in control for as long as you want to be.

Your diet stands a miles better chance of success, if you don't fill yourself with fatty, salty or sugary foods, the weight stands a huge chance of dropping off without doing much else at all.

You can look yourself in the eye again.

You won't sabotage your health with these foods *ever again*.

NOTE 1: HOW MANY CALORIES WILL YOU SAVE?

I wonder exactly how many calories you will save from not eating the 3 small packets of crisps a day that I used to eat, let's see:

Take a look at this!

1 small packet is around 130 to 160 per 25g pack (or 560kj) depending on the type, ridged ones are highest in calories.

I used to get through at least 3 a day, often more but we'll say 3 small packets :
That's 140 x 3 calories per day = 420 calories per day just in crisps.

The 3 small packets of crisps a day comes out at a total of 2,940 calories per week, times 52 weeks = 152,880 calories in one year.

This has got to be a variable figure but it is a good guide.
I haven't counted my calories but I lost a stone in 4 months and not having done anything except ditch the crisps. Actually I kept on losing weight, more slowly but it went all the same. With exercise thrown in, I'm just over 2 stone less now!

So there it is, it will work if you do it. You can no doubt see why I put the warnings up not to read if you don't truly mean to do this , because even just the thought of it could spoil you for that food until it wore off.

Note 2: Can I Change Back If I Want To?

Yes. Don't worry, it will wear off unless you work on it from time to time. It may take a while if you have done a good job, but it will go eventually if you don't do the Click Click.

If you visualise strongly enough and <u>do it every single time</u> that temptation comes your way, Click, Click, you will conquer this I promise you. And after a while you simply won't even be tempted anyway.

Congratulations!

All the best,

Sophie Johnson

PS: Want To See How I Look Now?

Sophie Johnson

Here I come! Free of crisps and slim enough for a woman of my age, not too shabby for a pensioner, well I think so anyway.

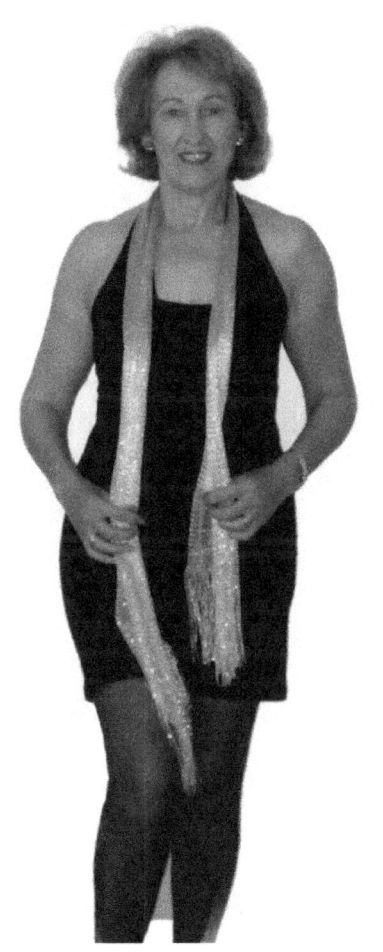

Yep! I did do it myself, no crisps, I never even think about it now and of course no fat!

You can do it too!

Sophie.

You can email me with your story on:

publishonamazon@gmail.com

or visit my website at: www.PublishonAmazon.co.uk

if you have an idea for a book of your own.